WEIGHT LOSS RECIPES COOKBOOK

"Delicious and Healthy Meals to Help You Shed the Pounds!"

Luna Roy

Copyright © [2023] [Luna Roy]

TABLE OF CONTENT

INTRODUCTION

Carolina had been trying for years to lose weight, but nothing seemed to work. She had tried any diet she could find, but the results were minimal at best. She was growing impatient with her lack of progress.

One day while looking online, she stumbled upon one of my articles about how to lose weight with the right diet and some other useful information.

The diet consisted of eating a balanced and nutritious meal plan with plenty of vegetables and protein. She was motivated to give it a try.

Carolina started tracking her meals and sticking to her meal plan. She was surprised to find how easy it was to stick to her new routine

In just a few months, Carolina had lost several pounds. She felt better than ever before and was able to finally fit into her favorite dress.

Carolina continued to stay on the diet and was able to maintain her new, healthier lifestyle.

She kept up with regular exercise and continued to eat balanced meals. Carolina was finally at her goal weight and felt amazing. She could not believe that all she needed was the right diet and it had made all the difference.

She now had a newfound confidence and was happy with her new lifestyle.

Weight loss is a journey of hard work, dedication, and determination. It's an ever-changing path that can lead you to improved physical and mental health. With the right plan and a little motivation, you can unlock the key to a healthier and happier you. Now is your time to take the first step toward the body and life you've always wanted.

Gone are the fad diets or crazy exercise routines. Weight loss comes down to a few simple principles — reducing calorie intake, increasing physical activity, and adopting healthy habits. In the pursuit of a healthy lifestyle, a combination of nutrition planning, tracking progress, and staying mindful of your goals drives success.

Most importantly, by believing in yourself and committing to your health and well-being, you create a sustainable and life-long journey of weight loss that is both rewarding.

This is your opportunity to start a new and fulfilling path. So why wait? Let's take the first step towards a healthier and more successful you.

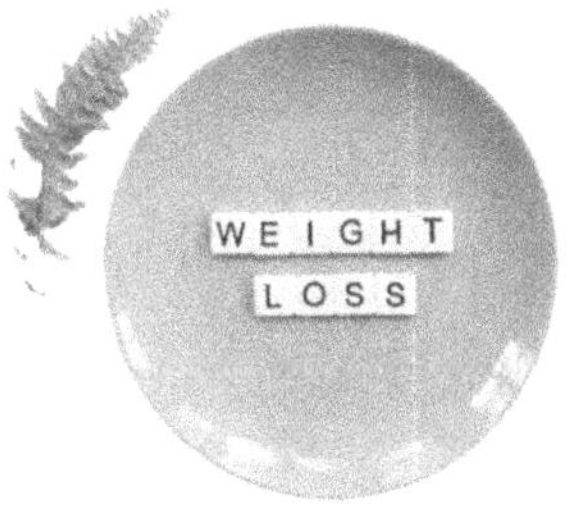

CHAPTER 1

Getting Started with a Healthy Lifestyle

One of the greatest challenges faced by many people today is weight loss. It can be difficult to reach and maintain a healthy weight for many people. Fortunately, weight loss success is achievable for those willing to embrace a healthy lifestyle.

Possible Causes of Weight Loss

Weight gain is a complicated issue with numerous possible causes. Although a healthy, balanced diet and regular exercise are the cornerstones of maintaining a healthy weight, many conditions and factors can contribute to excessive weight gain.

Common causes of weight gain include lifestyle choices, lack of physical activity, physiological and psychological conditions, hormonal changes, and certain medications.

In addition, age, genetics, and environmental factors can all play a role in the development of weight gain.

1. **Lifestyle choices** – Unhealthy eating habits, such as eating large amounts of processed and fast foods and consuming excessive amounts of sugar, fat, and carbohydrates, can all contribute to excessive weight gain. Additionally, a sedentary lifestyle with a lack of physical activity can also lead to increased calorie intake and weight gain.

2. **Physiological and psychological conditions** –Certain medical conditions, such as hypothyroidism or polycystic ovarian syndrome, can cause hormonal imbalances that lead to weight gain. Additionally, stress, anxiety, and depression can lead to emotional eating and an increase in caloric intake, both of which can result in weight gain.

3. Hormonal changes –Hormonal changes in women, such as those that occur during menopause and perimenopause, can cause weight gain.

4. Certain medications – Certain medications, such as steroids, antidepressants, and hormonal contraceptives, can cause weight gain, as well as fluctuations in blood sugar levels and a decrease in the body's ability to metabolize fats.

5. Age – As we age, our metabolism slows down, leading to a decrease in the ability to burn calories.

6. Genetics – Genetics can play a role in weight gain, as certain genetic variations can influence body weight and fat distribution.

7. Environment –The food environment and the availability of healthy options can also contribute to excessive weight gain. People who live in communities with limited access to healthy foods are more likely to consume diets high in sugar and fat, leading to increased caloric intake and weight gain.

A healthy lifestyle means more than just eating healthy. It is about taking a balanced approach to health that includes physical activity, healthy eating, taking care of emotional well-being, and engaging in activities that bring joy. Here are some steps to help you on your journey to weight loss success through a healthy lifestyle

1. **Move your body**. Aerobic exercise like brisk walking, jogging, cycling, or swimming is essential for shedding excess fat. For best results, aim for at least 30 minutes of moderate physical activity five times a week.

2. **Watch what you eat**. Eating healthy isn't just about avoiding junk foods. You have to eat balanced, nutritious meals and snacks that are packed with essential nutrients. Avoid processed and refined foods when possible and focus on lean proteins, healthy fats, fruits, and veggies.

3. **Get plenty of rest**. Sleep is very imperative and essential for your physical and emotional well-being. Aim for eight hours of quality sleep every night, and add naps in if needed.

4. **Manage stress levels**. Stress can be a major impediment to achieving a healthy weight. When you feel overwhelmed, find healthy ways to manage stress such as journaling, practicing yoga or meditation, or talking with a therapist.

5. **Make time for fun**. Having fun is crucial to living a healthy lifestyle. Make time for activities that bring you joy, and try to do something you enjoy every day.

Adopting a healthy lifestyle is key to achieving successful weight loss. Taking small steps each day to move your body, eat nutritious meals, get enough rest, manage stress levels, and make time for fun will lead to long-term health benefits.

By committing to a healthy lifestyle, you can set yourself up for weight loss success that lasts long into the future.

CHAPTER 2

Meal Planning for Weight Loss

14 days of meal planning

Day 1

Breakfast: 2 boiled eggs, half an avocado, 1 slice of whole wheat toast

Lunch: Greek salad with chickpeas and feta

Snack: Celery sticks with hummus

Dinner: Grilled fish and roasted broccoli

Day 2

Breakfast: Smashed avocado toast with tomatoes and feta

Lunch: Turkey and spinach wrap

Snack: Apple slices with almond butter

Dinner: Roasted cauliflower and quinoa

Day 3

Breakfast: Protein smoothie with banana, peanut butter, and almond milk

Lunch: Grilled chicken with sautéed vegetables

Snack: Carrots and hummus

Dinner: Baked sweet potato with black beans and spinach

Day 4

Breakfast: Overnight oats with raspberries and walnuts

Lunch: Salmon poke bowl

Snack: Handful of nuts

Dinner: Zucchini noodles with grilled shrimp

Day 5

Breakfast: Spinach and mushroom omelette

Lunch: Lentil soup

Snack: Celery and peanut butter

Dinner: Grilled chicken with roasted Brussels sprouts

Day 6

Breakfast: Banana, kiwi, and spinach in a green smoothie

Lunch: Chickpea and feta wrap

Snack: Plain Greek yogurt with berries

Dinner: Quinoa and vegetable stir fry

Day 7

Breakfast: Peanut butter and banana toast

Lunch: Mediterranean salad with grilled tofu

Snack: Apple slices with almond butter

Dinner: Baked salmon with asparagus and roasted sweet potato

Day 8

Breakfast: Overnight oats with almond milk and chia seeds

Lunch: Chickpea and quinoa veggie burger

Snack: Celery sticks with hummus

Dinner: Roasted vegetables with grilled chicken

Day 9

Breakfast: Scrambled eggs with bell peppers and tomatoes

Lunch: Kale salad with grilled fish

Snack: Apple slices with peanut butter

Dinner: Avocado and black beans with baked sweet potatoes

Day 10

Breakfast: Protein smoothie with berries, banana, and almond milk

Lunch: Lentil soup

Snack: Handful of nuts

Dinner: Quinoa and vegetable stir fry

Day 11

Breakfast: Oatmeal with banana and almond milk

Lunch: Grilled chicken salad

Snack: Celery sticks with peanut butter

Dinner: Roasted cauliflower and quinoa

Day 12

Breakfast: Avocado toast with tomatoes and feta

Lunch: Turkey and spinach wrap

Snack: Apple slices with almond butter

Dinner: Zucchini noodles with grilled shrimp

Day 13

Breakfast: Greek yogurt with muesli and berries

Lunch: Mediterranean salad with grilled tofu

Snack: Handful of nuts

Dinner: Roasted sweet potato and asparagus with baked salmon

Day 14

Breakfast: Egg omelette with bell peppers and tomatoes

Lunch: Kale salad with grilled fish

Snack: Celery sticks with hummus

Dinner: Grilled chicken and roasted broccoli

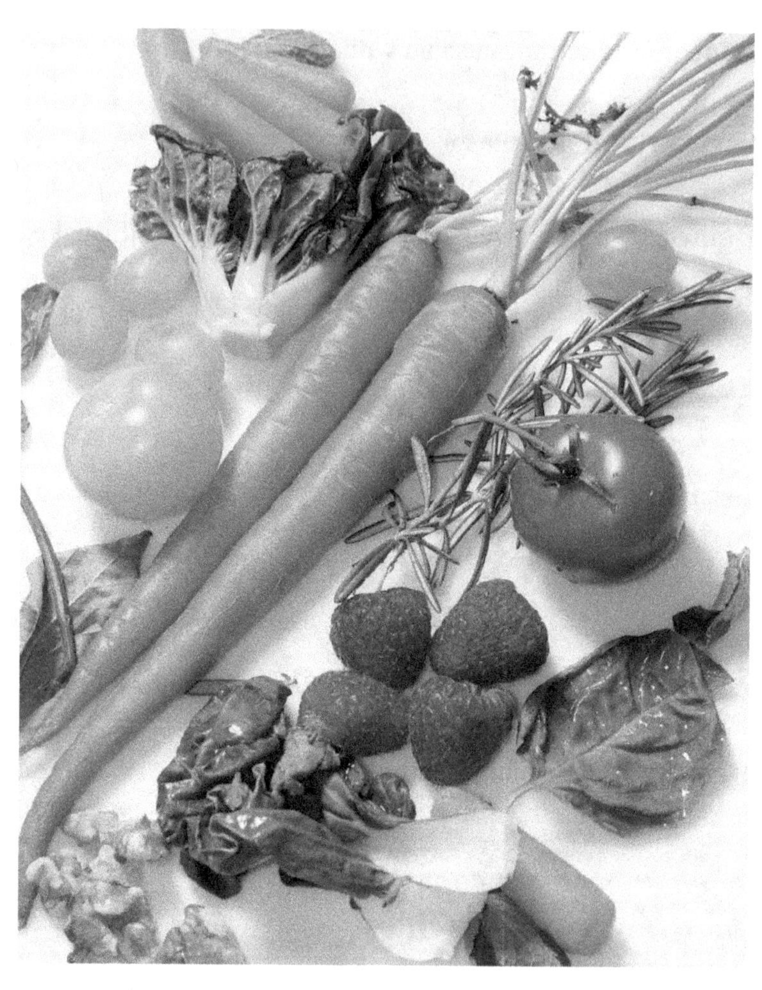

CHAPTER 3

Breakfast Recipes for Weight Loss

2 boiled eggs, half an avocado, 1 slice of whole wheat toast

Prep Time: 5 minutes

Ingredients:

-2 eggs

-1/2 of an avocado

-1 slice of whole wheat toast

Instructions:

1. Boil the two eggs for 3-5 minutes in a medium-sized pot with boiling water.

2. While the eggs are boiling, cut the avocado in half and gently remove the pit. Then slice each half lengthwise.

3. Toast the whole wheat bread in a toaster or on a pan on low-medium heat.

4. When the eggs have finished boiling, carefully remove them from the hot water and place them aside.

5. Plate the toast and avocado slices and top with the boiled eggs.

6. Enjoy!

Smashed Avocado Toast with Tomatoes and Feta

Prep Time: 10 minutes

Cook Time: 0 minutes

Total Time: 10 minutes

Serves: 1

Ingredients:

1 ripe avocado

2 slices of whole wheat toast

1/4 cup cherry tomatoes

1/4 cup crumbled feta cheese

Salt and pepper, to taste

Instructions:

1. Toast the bread slices in a toaster or a skillet on the stovetop.

2. Slice the avocado in half, remove the pit, and scoop from the skin. Place into a bowl and mash with a fork.

3. Apply the mashed avocado to the toast slices.

4. Top with cherry tomatoes and feta cheese.

5. Add salt and pepper to taste.

6. Serve and enjoy!

Overnight Oats with Raspberries and Walnuts

Prep Time: 5 minutes

Total Time: 8 hours 5 minutes

Servings: 2

Ingredients

• 2/3 cup old-fashioned rolled oats

• 1 teaspoon chia seeds

• 1 ½ cup non-dairy milk (almond milk, oat milk, etc.)

- 2 tablespoons maple syrup

- 2 tablespoons walnuts, chopped

- 1/3 cup raspberries, fresh or frozen

Instructions

1. In a medium bowl, mix the oats, chia seeds, non-dairy milk, and maple syrup.

2. Divide the oat mixture equally between two serving dishes.

3. Top each dish with walnuts and raspberries.

4. Cover the dishes and place them in the refrigerator to chill overnight.

5. Serve chilled and enjoy!

Greek Yogurt with Muesli and Berries

Prep Time: 10 minutes

Servings: 2

Ingredients:

• 2 cups Greek Yogurt

2 cups of muesli

• 1 cup of mixed berries (blueberries, raspberries, and blackberries)

• 2 tablespoons honey

• 2 tablespoons of toasted almonds, chopped

• 2 tablespoons of pumpkin seeds

Instructions:

1. Place the muesli in a mixing bowl and set aside.

2. In a separate bowl, combine the yogurt, honey, almonds, and pumpkin seeds. Mix ingredients thoroughly to ensure that they are all distributed equally.

3. In two individual bowls, divide the muesli mixture and top with the yogurt mixture.

4. Top the yogurt mixture with the mixed berries, then drizzle with honey (if desired).

5. Serve immediately and enjoy!

Oatmeal With Banana & Almond Milk

Cook Time: 10 minutes

Total Time: 15 minutes

Servings: 2

Ingredients:

• 2 cups almond milk

• 1 cup old-fashioned rolled oats

• 1 ripe banana, sliced

• 2 tablespoons honey (optional)

• 1 teaspoon ground cinnamon

Instructions:

1. Heat the almond milk in a medium saucepan over medium-high heat, stirring occasionally, until it comes to a gentle boil.

2. Add the oats and turn the heat to low.

3. Cook for about 10 minutes, stirring occasionally, until the oats are creamy and tender.

4. Divide the oatmeal into two bowls and top each with the banana slices, honey (if desired), and cinnamon. Serve immediately.

Scrambled Eggs with Bell Peppers and Tomatoes

Prep time: 10 minutes

Cook time: 10 minutes

Ingredients:

- 3 eggs

- 2 tablespoons butter

- ½ bell pepper, diced

- 2 Roma tomatoes, diced

- ½ teaspoon garlic powder

- ¼ teaspoon black pepper

- Salt, to taste

- 2 tablespoons chopped fresh parsley

Instructions:

1. Beat eggs in a bowl until well-combined

2. Heat butter in a non-stick pan over medium heat.

3. Add bell peppers and tomatoes to the pan and cook for 2 minutes.

4. Add garlic powder, black pepper, salt, and parsley. Stir and cook for 1 minute.

5. Add the beaten eggs to the pan and mix everything.

6. Cook for 4-5 minutes, stirring regularly, until eggs are cooked through.

7. Serve.

Peanut Butter and Banana Toast Recipe

Prep Time: 5 minutes

Cook Time: 5 minutes

Ingredients:

- 2 slices of whole wheat bread

- 2 tablespoons of creamy peanut butter

- 1 banana, thinly sliced

- Optional: honey, maple syrup, cinnamon

Instructions:

1. Preheat a toaster or toaster oven to medium heat.

2. Spread 1 tablespoon of peanut butter onto each bread slice.

3. Thinly slice 1 banana and lay the slices onto one of the bread slices.

4. Place the other bread slice on top of the banana slices.

5. Carefully place the sandwich in the toaster and toast for 4-5 minutes, until the bread is lightly golden and the peanut butter is melted.

6. Optional: For an extra touch of sweetness, add a drizzle of honey, maple syrup, or cinnamon on top of the toast.

7. Enjoy!

Overnight Oats with Almond Milk and Chia Seeds

Prep Time: 5 minutes

Cook Time: 8 hours

Ingredients

- ½ cup rolled oats

- ½ cup almond milk

- 2 tablespoons chia seeds

- 2 tablespoons honey

- ¼ teaspoon ground cinnamon

- ¼ teaspoon vanilla extract

Instructions

1. In a bowl or jar combine the rolled oats, almond milk, chia seeds, honey, cinnamon, and vanilla extract.

2. Stir to combine the ingredients until everything is evenly distributed.

3. Cover the bowl or jar and place it in the refrigerator overnight.

4. In the morning, remove the oats from the refrigerator and stir once more.

5. Serve cold or heat briefly in the microwave before consuming.

6. Enjoy!

Egg Omelette with Bell Peppers and Tomatoes

Prep Time: 10 minutes

Cook Time: 10 minutes

Total Time: 20 minutes

Ingredients:

-4 eggs

-2 bell peppers (chopped)

-1 tomato (diced)

-1/4 teaspoon of salt

-1/4 teaspoon of pepper

-3 tablespoons of olive oil

Instructions:

1. Heat a medium-sized skillet over medium heat.

2. Add the olive oil and let it heat up for a few minutes.

3. Add the bell peppers and tomato and cook for 2-3 minutes, stirring occasionally.

4. In a separate bowl, beat the eggs with the salt and pepper until combined.

5. Pour the egg mixture into the skillet, covering the vegetables.

6. Cook for 3-4 minutes until the eggs are cooked through.

7. Cook for a further 2 to 3 minutes after flipping the omelette.

8. Slice the omelette and serve. Enjoy!

Spinach and Mushroom Omelette

Prep Time: 10 minutes

Cook Time: 5 minutes

Total Time: 15 minutes

Servings: 1

Ingredients:

- 1 tablespoon olive oil

- 1/4 cup diced mushrooms

- 1/2 cup fresh baby spinach

- 2 large eggs

- 2 tablespoons milk

- Salt and pepper to taste

Instructions:

1. In a medium skillet, heat the oil over medium-high heat.

2. Add the mushrooms and sauté until tender, about 2 minutes.

3. Add the spinach and cook until wilted about 1 minute.

4. Whisk the eggs and milk together in a medium bowl.

5. Pour the egg mixture into the pan with the mushrooms and spinach and stir to combine.

6. Season with salt and pepper.

7. Cook until the eggs are cooked through, about 3 minutes.

8. Carefully flip the omelette and cook for an additional 1-2 minutes.

9. Serve hot. Enjoy!

CHAPTER 4

Snack Recipes for Weight Loss
Celery sticks with hummus

Prep time: 5 minutes

Ingredients:

- Celery sticks

- Hummus

Instructions:

1. Prepare the hummus according to package instructions.

2. Cut the celery sticks into chunks or thin strips, depending on your preference.

3. Serve the hummus in a bowl with the celery sticks.

4. Enjoy!

Apple Slices with Almond Butter

Prep Time: 5 minutes

Ingredients:

-2 apples

-1/3 cup almond butter

-Honey (optional)

Instructions:

1. Slice the apples into wedges.

2. Spread the almond butter over the slices.

3. Drizzle some honey on top, if desired.

4. Serve and enjoy!

Plain Greek Yogurt with Berries

Prep Time: 10 minutes

Ingredients:

-1 cup plain Greek yogurt

-1/2 cup fresh or frozen berries

-1 tablespoon honey (optional)

Instructions:

1. In a bowl, add the plain Greek yogurt and honey (if desired).

2. Mix the ingredients until blended.

3. Add the fresh or frozen berries to the yogurt and mix.

4. Serve as desired. Enjoy!

Carrots and Hummus

Prep Time: 10 minutes

Servings: 4

Ingredients:

- 8-10 carrots

- 1 cup hummus

- 2 tablespoons olive oil

- 2 cloves garlic, minced

- Juice of 1 lemon

- 1 teaspoon cumin

- Pinch of salt and pepper

Instructions:

1. Preheat oven to 400 degrees Fahrenheit.

2. Peel and dice carrots into 1/2-inch cubes.

3. Spread carrots onto a baking sheet lined with foil or parchment paper. Drizzle with olive oil and sprinkle with a little salt and pepper.

4. Roast for fifteen to twenty minutes or until fork-tender.

5. When carrots are done, let them cool slightly before transferring them to a bowl.

6. Whisk together hummus, garlic, lemon juice, and cumin in a small bowl.

7. Pour the hummus mixture over the carrots and stir until combined.

8. Serve immediately as is or with your favorite dipping sauces. Enjoy!

Handful of nuts

Prep time: 5min

1. **Ingredients:**

-3/4 cup of your favorite type of nuts (almonds, cashews, walnuts, etc.)

- 2 tablespoons of extra-virgin olive oil

-1 teaspoon of sea salt

-1 teaspoon of dried herbs such as oregano and thyme

Instructions:

1. Preheat oven to 350°F.

2. Spread the nuts out over a baking sheet covered with parchment paper.

3. Drizzle olive oil over the nuts and spread them out evenly on the baking sheet.

4. Sprinkle salt and herbs on top of the nuts.

5. Bake in the oven for about 10 minutes, stirring occasionally to make sure they are evenly toasted.

6. Let cool for a few minutes.

7. Enjoy your handful of nuts!

Apple slices with peanut butter

Ingredients:

2 Apples

2 Tbsp. Peanut Butter

Prep Time: 5 minutes

Instructions:

1. Wash and cut the apples into thin slices.

2. Spread peanut butter onto a plate.

3. Dip the apple slices into the peanut butter, making sure to coat both sides.

4. Enjoy!

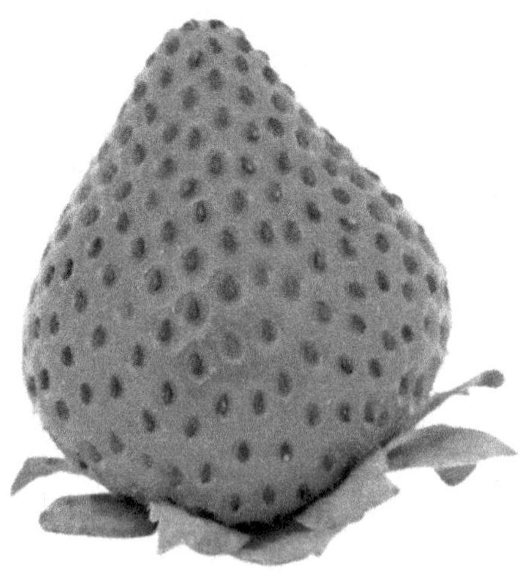

CHAPTER 5

Lunch Recipes for Weight Loss

Greek Salad with Chick Peas and Feta

Prep Time: 15 minutes

Servings: 4

Ingredients:

• 2 cups chopped romaine lettuce

• 1 cup sliced cucumber

• 1 cup cooked chickpeas

• 1/2 cup crumbled feta cheese

• 6 cherry tomatoes, quartered

- 1/4 cup sliced red onions

- 2 tablespoons extra virgin olive oil

- 1 tablespoon lemon juice

- 1 tablespoon dried oregano

- Salt and pepper to taste

Instructions:

1. In a large bowl, combine the lettuce, cucumber, chickpeas, feta, tomatoes, and onions.

2. In a small bowl, whisk together the olive oil, lemon juice, oregano, salt, and pepper.

3. Pour the dressing over the salad and toss until well combined. Serve immediately.

Turkey and Spinach Wrap

Prep Time: 15 minutes

Ingredients:

- 4 whole-wheat tortillas

- 1 lb. cooked turkey deli meat, sliced thin

- 2 cups baby spinach

- 1/4 cup salsa

- 1/2 avocado, sliced

Instructions:

1. Lay out your four whole-wheat tortillas on a clean flat surface.

2. Divide the turkey deli meat evenly and place on top of each of the tortillas.

3. Place the baby spinach on top of the turkey.

4. Drizzle the salsa over the spinach.

5. Place the sliced avocado on top of the salsa/spinach mixture.

6. Starting with the top of the tortilla, roll it up, tucking in the sides as you go.

7. Slice each wrap in half and serve. Enjoy!

Grilled Chicken with Sauteed Vegetables

Prep time: 10 minutes

Cook time: 30 minutes

Total time: 40 minutes

Ingredients:

- 2 boneless, skinless chicken breasts (4 ounces each)

- 2 teaspoons vegetable oil

- 1/2 cup chopped onions

- 1/2 cup chopped bell peppers

- 2 cloves garlic, minced

- 1/2 teaspoon dried basil

- 1/2 teaspoon dried oregano

- Salt and pepper, to taste

Instructions:

1. Preheat the grill to medium-high heat.

2. Rub the chicken breasts with the oil and season liberally with salt and pepper.

3. Grill the chicken for approximately 15 minutes per side.

4. While the chicken is cooking, heat a large skillet over medium heat.

5. Add the onions, bell peppers, garlic, basil, oregano, and a pinch of salt and pepper to the skillet and cook, stirring often, for about 5 minutes or until vegetables are just beginning to soften.

6. Once the chicken is cooked through, remove it from the grill and let rest for 5 minutes before slicing it into

Mediterranean Lentil Soup

Prep Time: 15 minutes

Cook Time: 45 minutes

Ingredients:

- 1 tablespoon olive oil

- 1 onion, chopped

- 2 cloves garlic, minced

- 2 carrots, chopped

- 1/2 cup celery, chopped

- 1 red bell pepper, diced

- 2 tablespoons tomato paste

- 1 teaspoon dried oregano

- 2 teaspoons ground cumin

- 4 cups vegetable broth

- 1 cup dry lentils

- 1/4 teaspoon cayenne pepper

- 1/4 teaspoon freshly ground black pepper

- 2 tablespoons parsley, chopped

- 1 can (14.5 ounces) diced tomatoes

Instructions:

1. In a large pot over medium heat, warm up the olive oil. Add onion and garlic and cook until softened about three minutes.

2. Add carrots, celery, bell pepper, tomato paste, oregano, and cumin. Stir to combine and cook for 5 minutes, or until vegetables are softened.

3. Pour in vegetable broth and lentils and add cayenne and black pepper.

4. Bring to a boil, then reduce heat to low and simmer for 30 minutes, or until lentils are tender.

5. Stir in diced tomatoes and cook for 5 more minutes.

6. Add parsley and serve. Enjoy!

Salmon Poke Bowl

Prep time: 25 minutes

Ingredients

- 2 cups of cooked and cooled sushi rice

- 2 tablespoons of sesame oil

- 1 pound of fresh, raw wild-caught salmon, cut into cubes

- 2 tablespoons of soy sauce

- 1 tablespoon of rice vinegar

- 1 teaspoon of freshly grated ginger

- 1 teaspoon of sesame seeds

- 1/2 teaspoon of seaweed furikake

- Sliced cucumbers, diced avocados, and sliced radish, for serving

Instructions

1. Start by preparing the sushi rice. Cook following the instructions on the package, and let the cooked rice cool completely.

2. Prepare the marinade for the salmon by combining the sesame oil, soy sauce, rice vinegar, ginger, sesame seeds, and furikake in a bowl and mix until well combined.

3. Add the salmon cubes to the marinade and let it sit for 15 minutes.

4. To assemble the poke bowl, divide the cooled sushi rice into individual bowls. Layer the marinated salmon over the rice and top with cucumbers, avocados, and radishes.

5. Enjoy your poke bowl!

Veggie Burger with Chickpeas and Quinoa

Prep Time: 15 minutes

Cook Time: 15 minutes

Servings: 4

Ingredients:

- 1 can chickpeas (drained and rinsed)

- 1 cup cooked quinoa

- 1 small onion (minced)

- 2 cloves garlic (minced)

- 1/2 cup breadcrumbs

- 1 egg

• 2 tablespoons olive oil

• 1 teaspoon ground cumin

• Salt and pepper to taste

• 4 hamburger buns

• Toppings such as lettuce, tomato, pickles, mayonnaise, mustard, etc.

Instructions:

1. Preheat the oven to 350°F. Prepare a baking sheet with parchment paper and set aside.

2. Place the chickpeas in a bowl and mash them using a fork until they are in small pieces.

3. Add the cooked quinoa, minced onion, minced garlic, breadcrumbs, egg, olive oil, cumin, and salt and pepper to the mashed chickpeas.

4. Mix the ingredients until everything is well combined.

5. Form the mixture into four patties and place them on the prepared baking sheet.

6. Bake the patties in the preheated oven for 15 to 20 minutes until they are golden brown and crispy.

7. Serve the veggie burgers on hamburger buns with your desired toppings. Enjoy!

Kale Salad with Grilled Fish

Prep Time: 10 minutes

Cook Time: 10 minutes

Total Time: 20 minutes

Ingredients:

- 2 bunches of kale, washed and chopped

- 2 tablespoons olive oil

- 2 cloves garlic, minced

- 2 tablespoons balsamic vinegar

- 2 teaspoons honey

- Salt and pepper, to taste

- 2 salmon filets

- 2 tablespoons butter, melted

Instructions:

1. Preheat your grill to medium-high heat.

2. In a large bowl, combine the kale, olive oil, garlic, balsamic vinegar, honey, salt, and pepper. Mix until everything is combined.

3. Place the salmon filets onto the grill and brush them with melted butter. Grill each side for 5-7 minutes, or until thoroughly cooked

4. Plate the kale salad and top with the grilled salmon. Enjoy!

Grilled Tofu Mediterranean Salad

Prep Time: 10 minutes

Cook Time: 4 minutes

Total Time: 14 minutes

Ingredients:

-1/2 lb. firm tofu, cut into cubes

-1/4 cup olive oil

-2 garlic cloves, minced

-1/2 teaspoon dried oregano

-Salt and pepper to taste

-1/4 cup red wine vinegar

-1 can dice tomatoes

-1 red onion, chopped

-1 cucumber, diced

-1 bell pepper, diced

-1/4 cup chopped fresh parsley

-1/4 cup crumbled feta cheese

Instructions

1. Preheat the grill to medium-high heat.

2. In a small bowl, mix the olive oil, garlic, oregano, salt, and pepper. Brush the mixture onto the cubes of tofu.

3. Grill the tofu for about 4 minutes, turning occasionally, until lightly charred and cooked through.

4. In a large bowl, combine the cooked tofu, tomatoes, red onion, cucumber, bell pepper, parsley, feta cheese, and red wine vinegar.

5. Toss lightly to combine and season with additional salt and pepper if desired.

6. Serve immediately and enjoy!

Grilled chicken salad

Total Prep Time: 15 minutes

Ingredients:

-2 boneless, skinless chicken breasts

-2 tablespoons olive oil

-Salt and pepper

-1 cup grape tomatoes, halved

-2 cups spinach

-1 cucumber, diced

-1/4 cup crumbled feta cheese

-1/4 cup balsamic vinaigrette

Instructions:

1. Preheat a grill to medium-high heat.

2. Rub the chicken with the olive oil, and season with salt and pepper.

3. Grill each side of the chicken for 5-7 minutes, until cooked through. Remove the grill and allow to cool.

4. In a large bowl, combine the tomatoes, spinach, cucumber, feta, and vinaigrette and mix.

5. Slice the chicken and add it to the salad.

6. Serve chilled or at room temperature. Enjoy!

Chickpea and Feta Wrap

Prep Time: 15 minutes

Ingredients

-1 (15-ounce) can of washed and drained chickpeas

-1/4 cup pesto

-1/4 cup crumbled feta cheese

-1/4 cup chopped red onion

-1/4 cup diced tomatoes

-4 (10-inch) gluten-free tortillas

Instructions

1. In a medium bowl, mash chickpeas with a fork or masher.

2. Stir in pesto, feta cheese, red onion, and tomatoes.

3. Take a tortilla and spread a portion of the chickpea mixture onto one-half of the wrap.

4. Fold the other half of the wrap over the filling and press lightly.

5. Repeat with the leftover tortillas and filling.

6. Heat a non-stick skillet on medium-high heat and place the wrap on the skillet.

7. Cook for 2-3 minutes or until lightly golden brown.

8. Flip it over, then repeat on the other side.

9. Serve warm with your favorite sides. Enjoy!

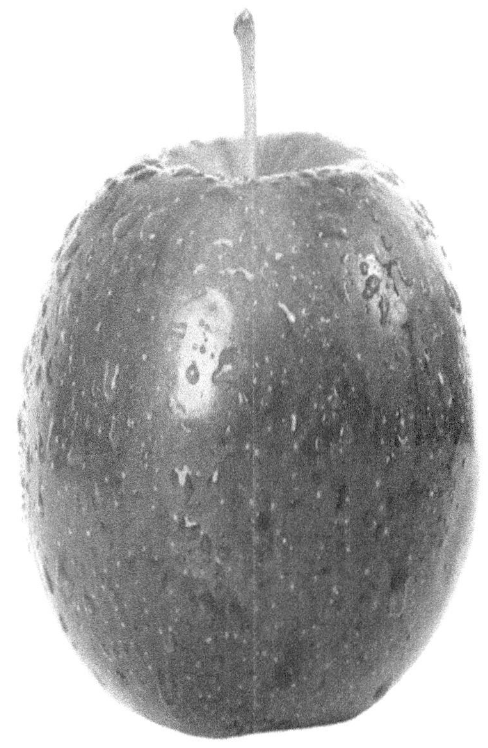

CHAPTER 6

Dinner Recipes for Weight Loss Grilled Fish and Roasted Broccoli

Prep Time: 10 minutes

Cook Time: 25 minutes

Total Time: 35 minutes

Serves: 4

Ingredients:

4-6 fillets of whitefish such as cod, tilapia, or bass, deboned

2 tablespoons of olive oil

1 teaspoon of garlic powder

1/2 teaspoon of salt

1/4 teaspoon of ground black pepper

1 substantial head of broccoli, cut into florets

2 tablespoons of olive oil

1/2 teaspoon of garlic powder

1/4 teaspoon of sea salt

Instructions:

1. Set the oven to 400 degrees F (204 C).

2. Pat the fish fillets dry with a paper towel, then brush each side lightly with olive oil and season with garlic powder, salt, and pepper. Set aside.

3. Place the broccoli florets onto a baking sheet and drizzle with olive oil. Sprinkle with garlic powder and sea salt. Mix to coat the florets.

4. Place the baking sheet in preheated oven and roast for 15 minutes.

5. Meanwhile, preheat a large skillet over medium-high temperature. Add the fish fillets and cook for 3-4 minutes per side or until the fish is golden brown and cooked through.

6. Remove the baking sheet from the oven and serve the grilled fish and roasted broccoli together. Enjoy!

Roasted Cauliflower and Quinoa

Prep Time: 10 minutes

Cook Time: 25 minutes

Total Time: 35 minutes

Serves: 4-6

Ingredients:

- one head of cauliflower, cut into small florets

-1 cup of quinoa

-1/4 cup of olive oil

-2 tablespoons of lemon juice

-1 teaspoon of garlic powder

-1 teaspoon of onion powder

-1/2 teaspoon of paprika

-Sea salt and black pepper to taste

Instructions;

1. Set your oven to 400 degrees F and line a baking sheet with parchment paper.

2. In a large bowl, combine the cauliflower florets, quinoa, olive oil, lemon juice, garlic powder, onion powder, paprika, sea salt, and black pepper to taste. Mix everything togel evenly coat.

3. Spread the mixture evenly onto the parchment paper-lined baking sheet.

4. Roast in the preheated oven for 20-25 minutes, or until the cauliflower is tender and golden brown and the quinoa is cooked through.

5. Serve warm or at room temperature. Enjoy!

Grilled Shrimp and Zucchini Noodles

Prep Time: 20 minutes

Cook Time: 10 minutes

Total Time: 30 minutes

Ingredients:

- 2 zucchinis

- 12-16 ounces of peeled and deveined shrimp

- 2 tablespoons extra virgin olive oil

- 2 tablespoons chopped fresh herbs (e.g. parsley, basil, or oregano)

- 2 cloves garlic, minced

- Juice from one lemon

- Salt and pepper, to taste

Instructions:

1. Preheat a grill or grill pan over medium-high temperature.

2. Use a spiralizer or julienne peeler to create zucchini noodles. Put in a sizeable bowl, then set aside.

3. In a smaller bowl, combine olive oil, herbs, garlic, lemon juice, salt and pepper.

4. Thread the shrimp onto skewers.

5. Brush the shrimp skewers on both sides with the herb mixture.

6. Grill the shrimp for 4-6 minutes, turning once halfway through, until cooked through.

7. Add the cooked shrimp to the bowl with the zucchini noodles and pour any remaining herb mixture over top.

8. Toss to combine.

9. Serve warm. Enjoy!

Baked Sweet Potato with Spinach and Black Beans

Prep Time: 10 minutes

Cook Time: 40 minutes

Total Time: 50 minutes

Ingredients:

• 2 large sweet potatoes, cleaned and sliced into wedges

• 1 tablespoon olive oil

• 1 teaspoon of garlic powder

• 1 teaspoon of chili powder

• one can of washed and drained black beans

• one cup of spinach, washed and chopped

• 1 teaspoon of cumin

Instructions:

1. Set the oven to 400 degrees Fahrenheit.

2. Place the sweet potatoes on a baking sheet with olive oil drizzled over them.

3. Sprinkle garlic powder, chili powder, and cumin onto the potatoes.

4. Bake for 20 minutes.

5. Turn the potatoes over and bake for an additional 20 minutes.

6. Meanwhile, heat the black beans with the spinach in a saucepan over medium-high heat for 5-7 minutes.

7. To serve, divide the sweet potatoes between two plates and top with the black beans and spinach mixture.

Enjoy!

Grilled Chicken with Roasted Brussels Sprouts

Prep Time: 25 minutes

Ingredients:

- a pound of skinless, boneless chicken breasts

- 1 pound Brussels sprouts

- 2 tablespoons olive oil

- Salt and pepper to taste

Instructions:

1. Preheat your oven to 375 degrees.

2. Wash the Brussels sprouts and discard any bad or wilted leaves. Cut the Brussels sprouts in half.

3. Place the Brussels sprouts in a large bowl or on a sheet pan. Add the olive oil and season with salt and pepper. Mix the Brussels sprouts to coat evenly in the oil.

4. Place the Brussels sprouts in the oven and roast for about 18 minutes, or until they are golden and slightly charred.

5. While the Brussels sprouts are in the oven, season the chicken breasts with salt and pepper on both sides.

6. Heat a grill pan over medium-high heat. Once the pan is hot, add the chicken breasts and cook for 6-7 minutes per side, or until they are cooked through and golden brown.

7. Once the Brussels sprouts and chicken are cooked, place them on a plate and serve. Enjoy!

Quinoa and Vegetable Stir Fry

Prep Time: 10 minutes

Cook Time: 10 minutes

Total: 20 minutes

Ingredients:

- 2 tablespoons of oil

- 2 cloves of garlic, minced

- 2 carrots, diced

- 1 red bell pepper, diced

- ⅓ cup of frozen peas

- 2 tablespoons of soy sauce

- ½ teaspoon of ground ginger

- 2 cups of cooked quinoa

Instructions:

1. In a large skillet, warm the oil over medium heat

2. Add garlic and sauté for 1 minute, stirring constantly.

3. Add carrots, bell pepper, and peas to the skillet and cook for 3 minutes, stirring occasionally.

4. Add soy sauce and ginger and stir until combined.

5. Add cooked quinoa and stir to combine.

6. Cover and cook for five minutes, stirring occasionally.

7. Serve and enjoy!

Salmon Baked with Roasted Sweet Potatoes and Asparagus

Prep Time:15 minutes

Cook Time:20 minutes

Total Time:35 minutes

Ingredients:

- 4 salmon fillets

- 1 bunch of asparagus

- 2 sweet potatoes, peeled and cubed

- 2 tablespoons olive oil

- 2 tablespoons fresh lemon juice

- Sea salt and black pepper, to taste

- 3 cloves garlic, minced

- 2 tablespoons fresh chopped parsley

Instructions:

1. Preheat the oven to 375°F

2. Place the cubed sweet potatoes onto a baking sheet lined with parchment paper and drizzle them with 1 tablespoon of olive oil. Sprinkle with salt and pepper and toss everything together to combine. Roast in the oven for fifteen minutes.

3. While the sweet potatoes are roasting, prepare the salmon and asparagus. Place the salmon fillets onto a greased baking sheet and drizzle with 1 tablespoon of olive oil. Squeeze the lemon juice over the salmon and season with salt and pepper.

4. Place the asparagus onto another baking sheet lined with parchment paper and toss with the remaining olive oil, garlic, and parsley. Sprinkle with salt and pepper and mix to combine.

5. Place both pans in the oven and bake for 15-20 minutes, or until the asparagus and sweet potatoes are tender and the salmon has reached an internal temperature of 145 degrees Fahrenheit.

6. Serve the salmon, asparagus, and sweet potatoes together with fresh lemon wedges, if desired. Enjoy!

Roasted Vegetables and Grilled Chicken

Prep Time: 20 minutes

Cook Time: 30 minutes

Servings: 4

Ingredients:

- 2 sweet potatoes, cut into cubes

- 2 bell peppers, julienned

- 2 tablespoons olive oil

- 2 garlic cloves, minced

- ¼ teaspoon smoked paprika

- Salt and pepper, to taste

- 4 chicken breasts, boneless and skinless

- 2 tablespoons honey

- 2 tablespoons Dijon mustard

Instructions:

1. Preheat your oven to 375°F and line a baking sheet with aluminum foil.

2. Place the sweet potatoes and bell peppers on the baking sheet and drizzle with the olive oil. Sprinkle with garlic, smoked paprika, salt, and pepper, to taste.

3. Roast in the preheated oven for 25-30 minutes, or until the vegetables are tender.

4. Meanwhile, season the chicken breasts with salt and pepper, to taste.

5. Heat a grill pan over medium-high heat. Place the chicken breasts on the pan and cook for 5-7 minutes per side, or until chicken is cooked through.

6. In a small bowl, whisk together the Dijon mustard and the honey.

7. Once the chicken is cooked, brush it with the honey-Dijon mixture.

8. Serve the roasted vegetables with the grilled chicken. Enjoy!

Baked Sweet Potato with Avocado and Black beans

Total Time: 45 minutes

Servings: 4

Ingredients:

-4 sweet potatoes

-1 15-ounce can of black beans, cleaned and drained

-½ cup salsa

-½ teaspoon cumin

-½ teaspoon chili powder

-1 avocado, diced

-1 lime, divided

Instructions:

1. Preheat the oven to 375°F.

2. Wrap each sweet potato with aluminum foil and place directly on the oven rack. Bake for 40 minutes.

3. Meanwhile, in a medium-sized bowl, combine the black beans, salsa, cumin, and chili powder. Set aside.

4. Peel and dice the avocado and squeeze the juice of ½ lime over it.

5. When the potatoes are finished, split the potatoes open lengthwise and top them with the black bean mixture.

6. Top with the diced avocado and squeeze the remaining lime juice over top.

7. Serve and enjoy!

Baked Lemon Herb Salmon with Steamed Asparagus

Prep Time: 10 minutes

Cook Time: 15 minutes

Ingredients:

- 1 pound salmon

- 2 tablespoons freshly squeezed lemon juice

- 2 tablespoons extra-virgin olive oil

- 2 tablespoons chopped fresh parsley

- 1 teaspoon fresh thyme

- Salt and pepper to taste

- 1 bunch of asparagus

Instructions:

1. Preheat oven to 375 degrees Fahrenheit.

2. Place salmon on a baking sheet and set aside.

3. In a small bowl, mix lemon juice, olive oil, parsley, thyme, salt, and pepper.

4. Spread the mixture evenly over the salmon.

5. Bake in the preheated oven for 10-15 minutes until the salmon is cooked through.

6. Meanwhile, prepare the asparagus. Begin by preparing a large pot of salted boiling water.

7. Once boiling, add asparagus to the pot and let cook for about 3-4 minutes until bright green and fork-tender.

8. Serve salmon with asparagus and enjoy!

CHAPTER 7

Dessert Recipes for Weight Loss

Grilled Peach with Greek Yogurt and Honey

Prep Time: 10 minutes

Cook Time: 10 minutes

Total Time: 20 minutes

Ingredients:

- 2 ripe peaches, halved and pitted

- 2 tablespoons olive oil

- 2 cups plain Greek yogurt

- Honey, for drizzling

- Fresh mint leaves, for garnish (optional)

Instructions:

1. Preheat a grill or grill pan to a medium-high setting

2. Brush the halved peaches with olive oil.

3. Grill the peaches for 5-7 minutes on each side, until softened and lightly charred.

4. Place the grilled peaches on a plate and top each half with Greek yogurt.

5. Drizzle with honey and garnish with fresh mint leaves, if desired. Enjoy!

Banana Oat Pancakes

Prep Time: 10 minutes

Cook Time: 10 minutes

Ingredients:

- 2/3 cup rolled oats

- 2 ripe bananas

- 1/4 teaspoon sea salt

- 2 tablespoons honey

- 2 teaspoons baking powder

- 1/2 cup milk

- 2 large eggs

- Two tablespoons and two teaspoons of melted butter

- 1 teaspoon vanilla extract

- 2 tablespoons vegetable or canola oil, for frying

Instructions:

1. In a blender or food processor, combine oats, bananas, salt, honey, baking powder, milk, eggs, butter, and vanilla and blend until smooth.

2. Over medium-low heat, preheat a heavy skillet or griddle. Add oil and let warm for 1 to 2 minutes.

3. Use a ladle to pour 1/4 cup of batter into the skillet. Cook for 2 minutes, or until the edges are lightly browned and the center of the pancake is slightly bubbly. Flip and cook for an additional one to two minutes.

4. Remove from the skillet and keep warm while preparing the remaining pancakes.

5. Serve pancakes

Dark Chocolate Bark

Prep time: 10 minutes

Cook time: 10 minutes

Yields: 8 servings

Ingredients:

• 12 ounces semisweet chocolate chips

• ½ cup toasted slivered almonds

• half cup of roasted and lightly salted peanuts

• ½ cup dried cranberries

• 1 teaspoon flaky sea salt

Instructions:

1. Set aside a baking sheet that has been lined with parchment paper

2. In a microwave-safe bowl, add chocolate chips and melt in the microwave for 1 minute. Stir the chips after each 30-second interval until melted.

3. Spread out the melted chocolate chips on the parchment-lined baking sheet, making sure to leave a border around the edges.

4. Sprinkle almonds, peanuts, cranberries, and sea salt evenly over the top of the chocolate.

5. Place the baking sheet into the refrigerator for 10 minutes, or until the chocolate has hardened.

6. Break the chocolate bark into pieces and enjoy!

Blueberry Sauce with Vanilla Ice Cream

Prep Time: 10 minutes

Ingredients:

- One and a half cups frozen or fresh blueberries

- 2 tablespoons granulated sugar

- 2 tablespoons water

- 2 tablespoons freshly squeezed lemon juice

- 2 tablespoons butter, melted

- 1 teaspoon cornstarch

- ¼ teaspoon ground cinnamon

- One pint of your preferred vanilla ice cream

Instructions:

1. In a medium saucepan, combine the blueberries, sugar, water, lemon juice, butter, cornstarch, and cinnamon.

2. Heat the mixture over medium heat, stirring constantly until it begins to boil.

3. Reduce the heat to low and allow the mixture to simmer for 5 minutes, stirring occasionally.

4. Remove the sauce from the heat and allow it to cool slightly.

5. Serve the blueberry sauce over a scoop of vanilla ice cream. Enjoy!

Chocolate Avocado Mousse

Prep Time: 10 minutes

Ingredients:

- 2 ripe avocados, pitted and peeled

- 1/3 cup pure maple syrup

- 1/2 cup cocoa powder

- 1 teaspoon vanilla extract

- 1/4 teaspoon ground cinnamon

- Pinch of sea salt

Instructions:

1. Place the avocado, maple syrup, cocoa powder, vanilla, cinnamon, and salt in a food processor.

2. Blend for 1-2 minutes, or until smooth and creamy.

3. Taste and adjust sweetness/flavors, if desired.

4. Transfer the mousse to individual bowls or a large bowl and chill in the refrigerator for 30 minutes before serving.

5. Serve chilled with fresh fruit, nuts, and/or chocolate shavings. Enjoy!

CHAPTER 8

Nourishing Beverages For Weight Loss

Honey-Lemon Water:

Introduction: Start your day with this light, refreshing, low-calorie, and metabolism-reviving drink.

Instructions: Take 1 cup of hot water and mix in 1 teaspoon of organic honey and the juice of 1/2 a lemon. Enjoy the honey after stirring until it dissolves

Ingredients:

-1 cup hot water

-1 teaspoon honey

-1/2 a lemon

Prep Time: 5 minutes

Detox Green Tea:

Introduction: This light, aromatic tea is full of antioxidants and nutrients, aiding in weight loss with its ability to help the body flush out toxins.

Instructions: Take 1 teaspoon of organic green tea leaves and steep in 1 cup of hot water for 5 minutes. Once brewed, add 1 teaspoon of organic honey and drink.

Ingredients:

-1 teaspoon organic green tea leaves

-1 cup of hot water

-1 teaspoon honey

Prep Time: 5 minutes

Apple Cinnamon Water:

Introduction: This sweet and spicy beverage tastes indulgent but is low in calories and features anti-inflammatory and antioxidant properties.

Instructions: Bring 1 cup of water to the boil and mix in 1/2 teaspoon of ground cinnamon. Take off the heat and add 1/4 cup of diced organic apples. Cover and allow to steep for 5 minutes, then strain and drink.

Ingredients:

-1 cup water

-1/2 teaspoon ground cinnamon

-1/4 cup diced organic apples

Prep Time: 10 minutes

Aloe Vera Juice:

Introduction: Aloe vera juice is packed with vitamins and minerals and has countless detoxification and weight-loss benefits.

Instructions: Take 1/2 cup of aloe vera juice and mix in a squeeze of fresh lemon juice and a teaspoon of organic honey. Stir to combine and drink.

Ingredients:

-1/2 cup aloe vera juice

-**Squeeze** fresh lemon juice

-1 teaspoon honey

Prep Time: 5 minutes

Detox Smoothie:

Introduction: This smoothie is full of vitamins, minerals, and antioxidants, and is dairy-free and full of good fats that support a healthy weight loss journey.

Instructions: Place 1/2 cup almond milk, 1/2 frozen banana, 1/4 cup frozen berries, 1 tablespoon of ground flaxseed, and 1 teaspoon of honey in a blender. Mix until smooth and creamy.

Ingredients:

-1/2 cup almond milk

-1/2 frozen banana

-1/4 cup frozen berries

-1 tablespoon ground flaxseed

-1 teaspoon honey

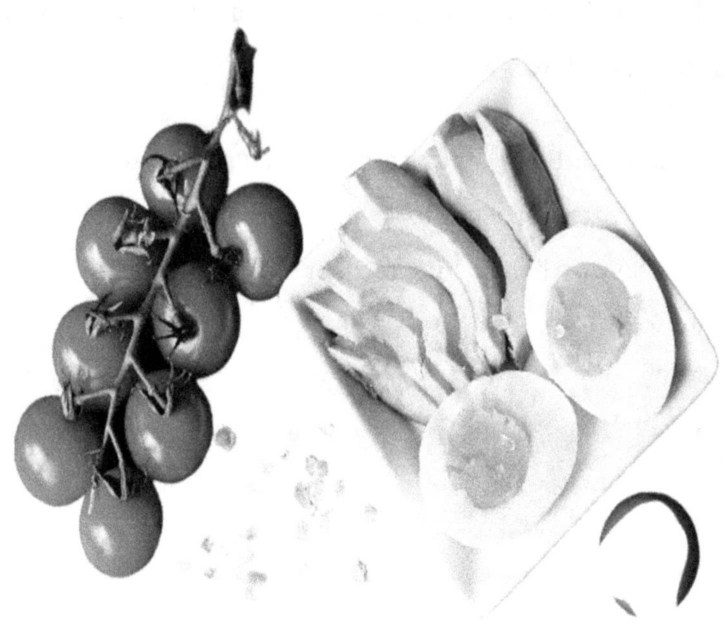

CHAPTER 9

Fitness and Exercise Tips for Weight Loss

Fitness and exercise are vital components of any successful weight loss program. Exercise helps to burn more calories and boost metabolism, while good nutrition helps to ensure that you are getting the right mix of nutrients to fuel your efforts. When combined, these two elements can result in significant and lasting weight loss. Here are some essential fitness and exercise tips for weight loss you should follow:

1. **Start Slow And Make Permanent Changes**: Take a realistic and gradual approach to fitness and exercise. A sudden, drastic change in either could take away from your progress. Start with a comfortable routine and slowly build up the intensity over time. Also, focus on behavior changes related to both nutrition and exercise that you can stick with for life.

2. **Change Up Your Routine**: You should always try to keep your workout routine fresh. Otherwise, you risk getting bored and losing motivation. You should also consider incorporating resistance training into your routine, as strength training helps to increase muscle mass and boosts metabolism.

3. **Find An Activity You Enjoy:** Exercise should not feel like a chore. Make sure to find an activity that you enjoy, as you will be more likely to stick with it over the long term. This could include anything from swimming to running to even simply taking a long walk.

4. **Make Exercise A Family Affair**: Exercise does not have to be something that you do solo. Consider finding ways to make exercise a family affair. This could involve playing a team sport or just going for a nature walk after dinner. By being active together, you will all be less likely to skip out on working out.

5. **Make Fitness Fit Into Your Lifestyle**: Exercise should not take up too much of your time. Consider finding ways to incorporate fitness into your regular daily routine. For example, take the stairs instead of the elevator or park further from the store and take a walk. If you incorporate fitness into your normal routine, it will be much easier to stick to it in the long run.

6. **Set Attainable Goals**: When it comes to reaching your fitness and exercise goals, make sure to find something that is realistic and attainable. Without a goal to shoot for, it will be all too easy for you to become discouraged and give up before you reach your desired weight loss. With that being said, make sure to celebrate your small successes along the way.

7. **Get Adequate Rest**: Make sure to get proper rest as it can have a major positive effect on your fitness and exercise progress. Not only will you be less tired while working out but you will be able to work at a higher level. Also, be sure to fuel your body properly post-workout to aid in recovery.

Exercises For Weight Loss

The role of fitness and exercise can not be undermined as a component of attainable weight loss programs. Here are a few examples of exercises that you can indulge yourself in;

1. **Aerobics**: Cardiovascular exercise, like running or swimming, burns calories and builds stamina, as well as reduces stress.

2. **Strength Training**: Strength training helps to build and maintain muscle mass, boost metabolism, and reduce body fat.

3. **Yoga**: Doing yoga can bring about several benefits for physical and mental health, such as better body awareness, a more flexible body, and improved breathing.

4. **Circuit Training**: Circuit Training is an intensive workout that combines strength and cardio exercises for an effective, full-body workout.

5. **Pilates**: Pilates is a form of exercise that uses specific movements and stretching techniques to help tone the body and improve overall strength.

Approximately 30 minutes of cardio exercise, three times per week, and two sessions of strength training per week are the basic guidelines for an effective weight-loss program.

Finally, consistency is key – make sure you choose an exercise routine that you can stick with regularly. Don't forget to eat a healthy diet and get enough rest, too. With these tips, you can be well on your way to achieving your weight-loss goals.

CHAPTER 10

Conclusion

At the end of the day, the goal of this cookbook has been to provide a range of recipes that are appropriate for those looking to make healthier food choices and to assist with weight loss. Any dietary plan, however, is only as good as its ability to fit into one's lifestyle. Every meal should be a balance of protein, carbohydrates, fats, vitamins, and minerals, all of which are essential for energy production and overall health.

In addition to the recipes provided, it is also important to focus on portion control. All of the recipes in this cookbook are designed to provide ample nutrition without overeating, which is often a core factor in weight loss. It is also a good idea to choose a variety of foods while cooking, and where possible to make meals from scratch using fresh ingredients.

Furthermore, it is important to plan. This book provides a well-defined 14 days meal plan which allows for portion control, meal varieties, and healthy food choices.

Having the right ingredients for your meal plan in your kitchen also eliminates the chance of poor food choices due to convenience and availability.

One of the most important tips we can give is to be consistent. Losing weight and maintaining a healthy weight doesn't happen overnight; Rome wasn't built in a day! Like any healthy habit, consistency is key to achieving the desired goal.

In conclusion, the recipes in the cookbook are just one part of the weight loss journey. Weight loss is a long-term process and requires dedication to achieve success. This cookbook can serve as a useful guide for those looking to make healthier food choices and assist with weight loss. With the right food choices, portion control, and consistent diet patterns, one is sure to see fruitful results.

I heartily wish you the best of luck in your journey toward a healthier you!